The Secret to a Healthy Pregnancy

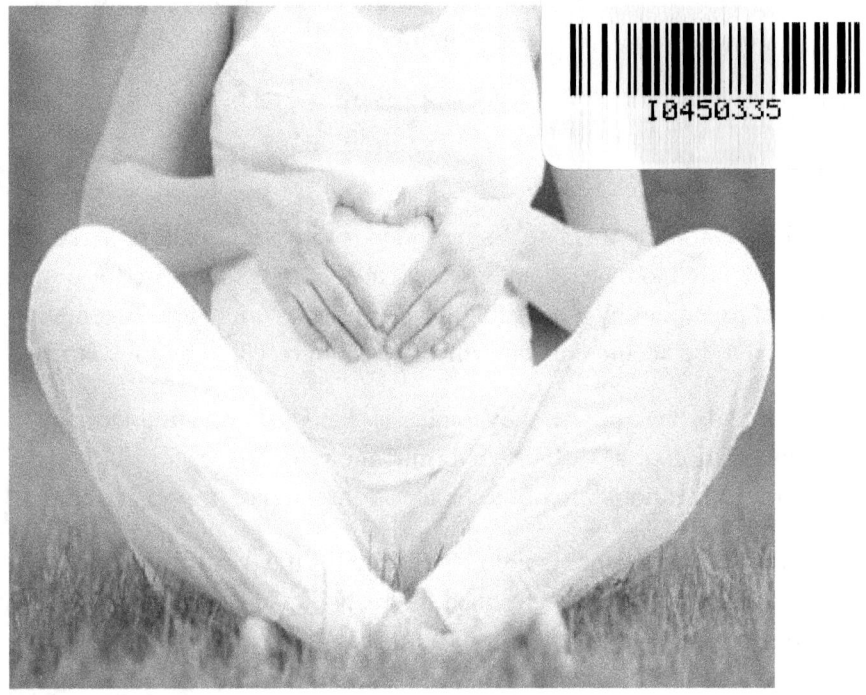

Health Learning Series

M. Usman

Mendon Cottage Books

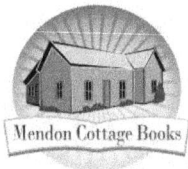

JD-Biz Publishing

Our books are available at

1. Amazon.com

2. Barnes and Noble

3. Itunes

4. Kobo

5. Smashwords

6. Google Play Books

Table of Contents

Introduction

Are you a mom to be? Congratulations! Your baby is indeed a blessing for you. But, his journey from heaven to earth is all in your belly. Your every act will affect your little new angel, including your habits, your attitude, and your routine. Don't panic on the fact you have to go through this alone. Also, don't be affright of all the advice given by the random ladies out there. Here we are just going to help you out in this crucial, as well as, blessed time.

This book covers almost each and every aspect of pregnancy. It reveals some secrets for the health of the charming angel in your hands. This book includes all the essential and basic steps you should take while you are expecting.

Put your hand on your belly and go through this book. You will end up having a joyous, healthy and fresh start with us.

Section 1: Nitty-Gritty of Your Blessed Life

You have wanted your own family. You might have coaxed the kids running and playing across the street. But, now you are going to have a pretty angel of your own in your lap. A storm of thoughts may have hit your mind if this is your first. But above all, this is going to be the most precious gift by your Lord. Through fervor, thrill and prevision, in the following chapters there is a lot more for you to discover and learn.

Chapter 1:10 Facts of Pregnancy

Pregnancy is one of the miracles of life. It totally changes your life from irresponsible crazy girl to a mature, responsible, and concerned mother. You are growing an individual all hidden inside your belly, isn't it incredible? You might have heard terrible stories of experiences by your friends of heart burn, sore breasts, hurting ankles or the longest wait of 9 months. But all this will be erased from your mind by the most precious gift of nature in your lap.

- A normal pregnancy is of 40 weeks (280 days) starting from the first day of your last menstrual period and is divided into three groups or trimesters, each of almost 3 months. .

- Most pregnancies last for 37 to 42 weeks. A newborn that comes in the world before 37 weeks is called premature or pre-term.

- The sex of the baby owes its appearance to floating sperms. It is the sperm from male that fertilizes the egg of the female and determines the sex of new comer.

- In the body of a female, a normal uterus grows bigger, approximately five hundred times its normal size during pregnancy. This change in size is for making space for the growing embryo.

- Early pregnancy symptoms involve missed periods, morning sickness, fatigue, breast tenderness and frequent urination.

- Pee stick pregnancy tests confirm pregnancy one week after the missed period. The test is positive due to the presence of a hormone called human chorionic gonadotropin hormone (HCG) in the urine. A blood test is more authentic and specific for the confirmation, but it takes time to confirm pregnancy.

- There is also weight gain of the body of a woman during pregnancy. Of the average weight gain, 40% of the weight is the baby.

- Progesterone height in your body softens the joints. For this you have to maintain a correct posture. Ligaments throughout the body, including the back, relax to an increase in hormone levels. Extra tension on the muscles of the back may cause pain.

- Every organ of the body shifts about to make a room for the new entry. The heart and liver grow in size due to the extra workload.

- In the end, you can thank your little new comer for the entire glow on your skin and healthy shiny crown of hair. The increased blood supply to the skin is responsible for the extra glow. High levels of estrogen and progesterone should be appreciated for a thick hairline.

Throughout pregnancy your baby grows in size from that of pinhead to 6 to 8 lbs. Normal range of the weight of the baby is between 6 pounds 2 ounces to 8 pounds. If you have decided to have all these facts for yourself then you are going to be the luckiest girl on the earth. You will be glad at each and every step of your expectancy period. You will be in the air for enjoying the feel of motherhood.

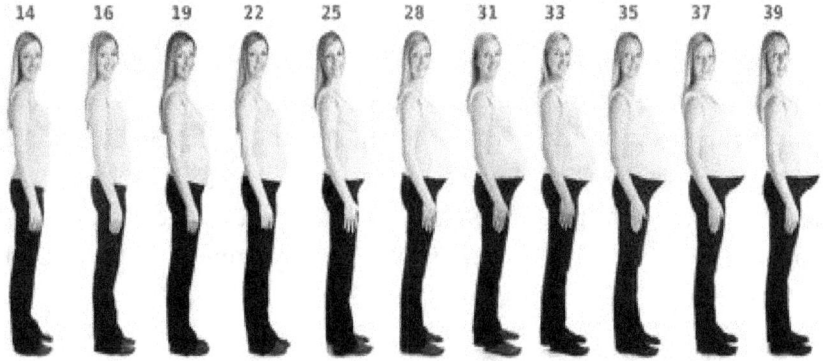

Chapter 2: Are You Expecting?

Pregnancy starts with some symptoms that are specific to each individual. This must be annoying for you to wait for the results to come or to keep checking for the early pregnancy symptoms. The following symptoms are crucial to pregnancy. If you have any of these alterations to your normal routine then you may possibly be pregnant.

Early pregnancy symptoms:

Early pregnancy symptoms are those which a woman experiences even when she is unaware of her pregnancy. Changes in the hormonal surge of estrogen, progesterone and HCG may cause early pregnancy symptoms. Some pregnancies stay asymptomatic for weeks or a month. Many moms to be find that during first month (before next periods) they feel nothing except tiredness.

- **A month without periods:**

Missed periods can throw a woman into panic, who used to have normal and regular menstrual periods. There can be a number of reasons for missed periods including your poor diet, certain medications causing disarray of hormones, or it can be the change of routine. But missed periods of pregnancy can be confirmed by a home pregnancy test (pee stick test) or a blood test. If these two beams strike you then it is a time to get prepared for good news.

- **Body temperature:**

Abrupt surge in progesterone levels can cause body temperature to remain elevated throughout pregnancy. If you are suspecting for pregnancy then keep check of your body temperature.

- **Morning with sickness:**

Another well known sign of pregnancy is morning sickness, which starts between 2 to 8 weeks after conception. It is not actually a morning sickness as it can attack you at noon or night with a full stomach. You may feel nauseated and it will end up with the expulsion of the stomach contents into the wash basin.

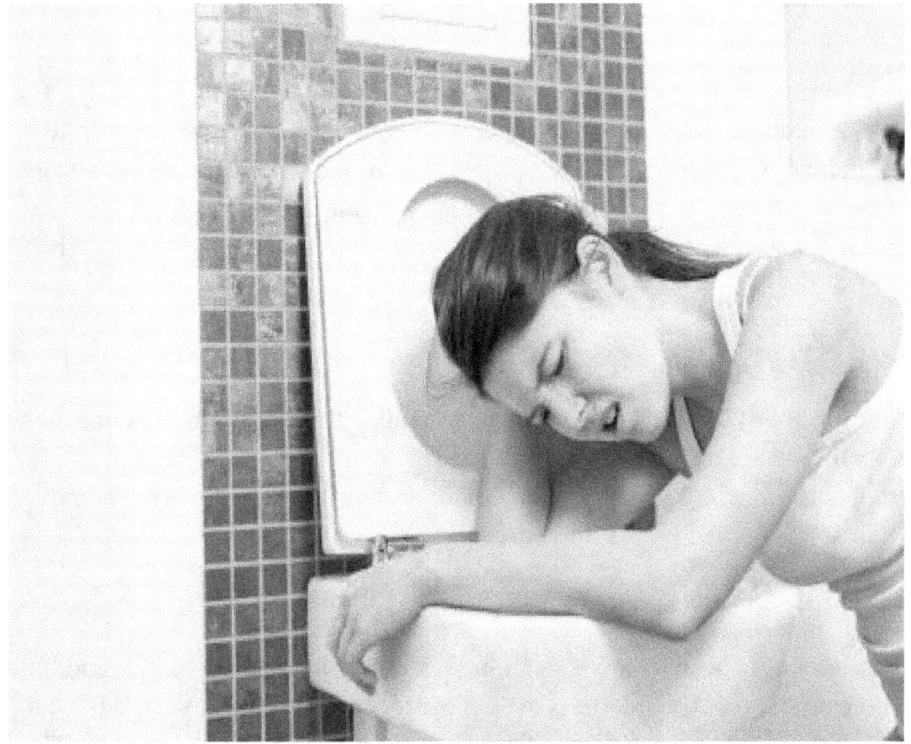

Late striking symptoms:

Once you have confirmed your pregnancy, the following chain of symptoms can strike. Don't get irritated at all these bad comings, as the end result of these is the prettiest thin in the world.

- **Fatigue:**

Feeling tired or burnt-out? It is normal for pregnancy. If you are exhausted all of a sudden, then surely it is due to the hormonal imbalance that is disturbing your body. For this, you just need to give time to your body and pamper it by keeping yourself well rested.

- **Shortness of breath:**

Out of breathe even without exertion? Don't blame your bones. You might be having a new soul hidden in your belly. This shortness of breath is due to location adjustment of breath organs making home for the new comer.

- **Vomiting and nausea:**

If you randomly fill your wash basin with your stomach contents, then it might be due to your pregnancy. This is because of high levels of estrogen and progesterone in the body quarrelling with the full stomach. This causes the stomach to empty more slowly and gives you a nauseated feeling when you eat.

- **Spotting:**

A little spot of blood on your under garments a few days before your regular menstrual date might be an indicator that you are expecting. This small amount of bleeding is due to the implantation of the baby embryo in his womb.

- **Breast tenderness:**

Swollen tingly bosoms are also an indicator of your starting motherhood. You can feel breast tenderness even during your menstrual cycle, but what makes this tenderness different from that of pregnancy, is its intensity. The strong soreness of breasts during pregnancy is due to a marked increase in female hormones (estrogen and progesterone). These hormones make increased blood supply to the breast, making them sensitive to the touch and painful. All of this is in the preparation of feeding breast.

- **Dizziness all the time:**

You have probably seen in movies, this go-to-symptom of fainting. This dramatic scene is created to signify pregnancy. It is not all in movies but it is a reality. Low levels of sugar or low blood pressure might be the culprit behind all this dizziness.

Section 2: Cramping First Trimester

Here we welcome you in the first stage of pregnancy, which is the first trimester. After you have confirmed your pregnancy with tests and all the above symptoms nettling you all the way, get prepared for the three hardest months of the first trimester. But, the torture of this trimester is a step to a holy change of status to the mother.

This section stores helping tips for you to cope through all the symptoms of first trimester. Stay calm and give it a read to unwrap the fitness secrets.

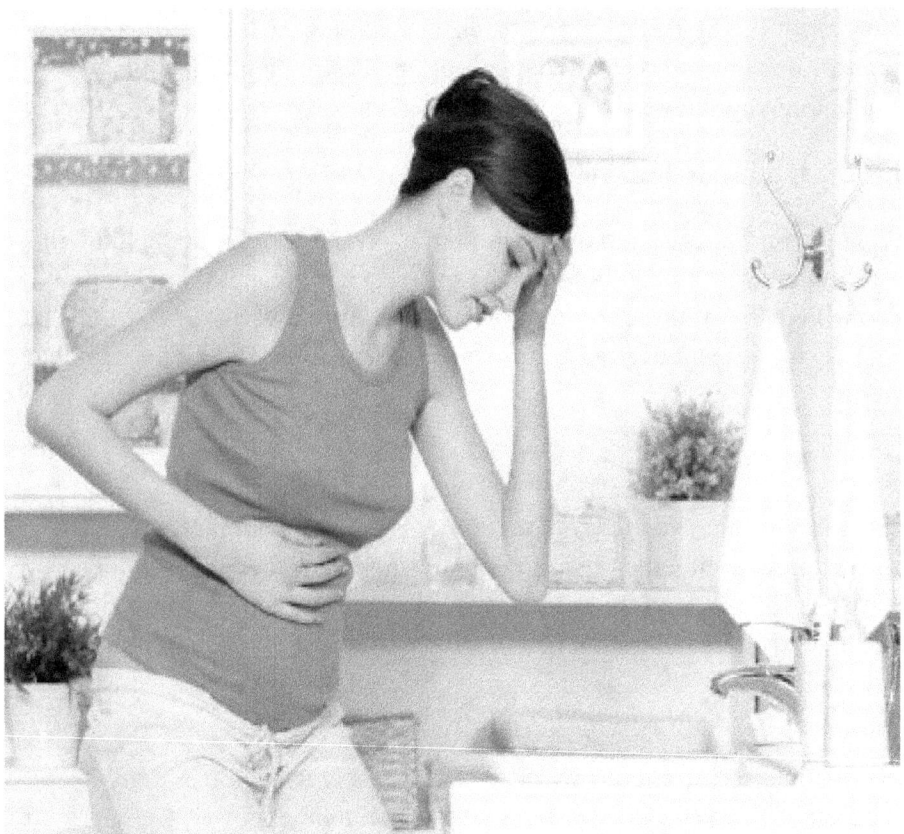

Chapter 1: Symptoms of the First 3 Months

The first 3 months, or the first trimester, starts from the first day of your last menstrual period. When the start of this trimester knocks at your door with good news, it brings some unwanted gifts for you as well. What the first trimester presents you also involves the early symptoms of pregnancy. Other blessings are as follow:

- **Cramping:**

Feeling cricks in your lower abdomen? Don't worry it is just normal for pregnancy. It may feel like same backache you have in your menstrual periods. It is due to your growing uterus and destruction of it walls by implanting your new baby.

- **Bathroom breakouts:**

When you have to rush to the washroom every 15 minutes, then you will surely curse your thought of having family. But relax, it is just temporary, you will get rid of these short journeys to washroom very soon. All this is because of pressure exerted on urinary bladder (urine bag) by the growing uterus.

- **Food appetence:**

If you have not craved for sour tamarind or you have not picked pickled mangos in your life, then this is the time when your food taste will avert to these tart foods. Go to the market and have some mouth-watering tangy pickles for your food aversion.

- **Super sense of smell:**

In this trimester, a pint of fragrance can be received by you as a dry heap. Pregnancy hormones kick your sense of smell to high power. Certain food smells can cause you to shun them. You may not like the smell of chicken or garlic. You may also cringe at the smell of certain perfumes.

- **Constipation:**

Producing waste will be a constant trouble for you from the start of the first trimester to the end of your pregnancy. This is because of the slow contraction of the muscles of the intestine. Pregnancy progesterone slows down the contracting muscles of the body.

- **Heart burn:**

Like the muscles of the intestine, the muscles of the esophagus and stomach also slow down. This causes the stomach food to run backward you're your esophagus instead of going to the end of your stomach. Entry of this food back into lower end of esophagus is called acid reflux or heart burn.

- **Mood swings:**

From the start of first trimester you will experience a roller coaster of emotions, making you cranky sometimes or terrified at others. Sometimes you will feel like crying. If this is the case then head for an understanding ear.

Chapter 2: Steps to Follow

Now that you have calmed down from the exciting news of getting pregnant, it is time to focus on the essential steps of care. You need to be very careful for the first three months of pregnancy, as your delicate baby is in the early stages of development. All the important organs of the baby are going to be formed during these months. Precautions should be taken at this time as to not disturb the developing baby. It is not that you need to sit stationed on a couch and watch television or live in a bubble. It is just that you should be well acknowledged and well prepared for the measures and precautions to be done.

- **Raise your demand of calories:**

Now your body needs your time and attention too. You will need to double your platter size with fresh and healthy food. Stock your kitchen with leafy green vegetables, fresh colorful juicy fruits, and meat. Take right and adequate quantities of food. Don't miss your meals.

- **Build up folic acid and iron stores:**

By the start of your pregnancy make sure you take iron and folic acid supplements on regular basis. Folic acid supplements should be started with the idea of getting pregnant as folic acid is required for the proper growth of your baby.

- **Keep snacks on hand:**

When you are expecting, your blood sugar can drop suddenly, making you dizzy. These symptoms can hit you during your work out. That is why you should keep snacks on hand at all times. This can be any sweet or mild chocolate or any fresh juice to get your sugar level up.

- **Get more sleep:**

Pregnancy hormones will make you exhausted. For this you have to take a few naps, whenever possible, to get back your energy. Your rest and sleep is very beneficial your baby. If you want your baby not to tease you at night, then get your sleep complete.

Exercise for your baby:

Regular mild exercise helps you to cope with the physical and mental changes that pregnancy brings to you. Exercise strengthens your muscle tone and pelvic floor. The key to fitness is to develop your habit slowly. The following exercises are considered safe for the first trimester:

- **Aerobics:**

Aerobics include brisk walking, mild running, and swimming. These exercises increase breathing and heart rate. These exertions improve body's use of oxygen and maintain the oxygen supply to your developing baby. Walking for 15 minutes daily can prevent you from varicose veins, fluid retention and hemorrhoids, which are dangerous for pregnancy. During the first trimester, swimming for at least 15 to 20 minutes three times a week will maintain a good shape for your figure

- **Yoga:**

Relax your mind and your muscles. Sit in a comfortable cool place, as over-heating is not good for the baby. Yoga, breathing, and relaxing exercises can stretch and improve your muscle tone. It relieves your stress and puts your body in the peace of mind and soul. These breathing techniques can also help you stay calm and focused during labor.

- **Pilates:**

Pilates is an excellent and amazing exercise to do during the first trimester of pregnancy. Pilates strengthens back muscles, maintains posture, and prevents back aches once you start gaining weight. Pilates may also enhance balance and stability by stretching all your body muscles. Pilates makes pelvic floor muscles strong to help with delivery. Continuing this technique after delivery helps to speed up weight loss after childbirth.

To deal with your morning sickness:

If you are tired of your nausea and vomiting all the time, then here is a simple tip for you. Try to take, small and frequent portions of meals to maintain adequate supply of calories. Don't grab warm sizzling food. Don't give your tongue oily spicy tastes. It will help you a lot. If you are facing a severe case then ask your care giver for some anti-emetics which are considered safe and effective for pregnancy.

- **Increase fluid intake:**

Vomiting and frequent urination can make you dehydrated, which is dangerous for your baby. Boost up your body with clean and clear water.

- **Work for your fatigue:**

It is necessary to listen to what your body tells you. For this, go easy on your household work. Share your work. Take frequent naps. Put your feet up whenever you feel you need to. Get a soothing massage to get relaxed.

- **Meet your midwife:**

Last but not the least; start searching for a good healthcare provider. Tell her all your concerns. Clear all your queries. Make a check of your blood group, blood pressure and all health details. Feel free to ask all your questions.

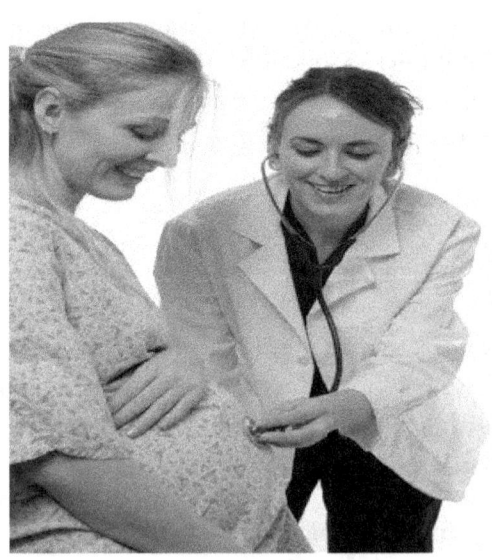

Chapter 3: Diet to Take

The secret to a healthy pregnancy lies in what you take in. If you want to enjoy your 9 month journey, you'll have to take good care of your diet. The health of your baby at the time of birth, owes its greater part to your diet and what you have selected during pregnancy. Furnish your refrigerator and kitchen with healthy and fresh items. For first trimester you have to adorn your dining table with folate rich food items for the developing nervous system of your baby. If your are feeling like gut-wrenching then grab some vitamin B6 to get rid of bad nausea and vomiting. We have formulated a diet plan for you, which you will enjoy sticking to.

- **Energizing breakfast:**

Take a glass of apple or cranberry juice. You can kick your energy with fruit smoothies, like a banana-berry smoothie, that will give you a power pack of 355 calories including proteins, calcium and vitamin C.

Add to your breakfast with high protein cereals made up of 1 cup skimmed milk and 2 tablespoon of almonds giving you 360 calories. You can also have scrambled eggs with toasted bread. Not going with your mood? Change it to yogurt with chopped slices of fruits like apricot, banana or apple.

- **Power pack snacks:**

Show your love for yogurt at brunch time. Slice some papaya and mix it with yogurt. You can also have a roll with peanut butter. This power pack will give you 150 calories.

- **Set a plate for lunch:**

Smoke some chicken and have it with some avocado salad. If not going with your mood, then have a baked potato with cottage cheese. Make sure you drink plenty of water. If you are bored with regular water, try adding some lemon or lime to it.

- **Another cracker:**

Garnish your supper with a handful of apricots. Add some almonds to it to get 290 calories. You can also have 1 to 2 handfuls of mixed nuts and dried fruits.

- **Kicking dinner:**

Make lamb chops with potatoes and peas. In your happy hours you can have your favorite macaroni and cheese pasta containing 340 calories.

Chapter 4: Don'ts of the Early Era

You have to familiarize yourself with some basic precautions from the first day of your expectancy period. These precautions are essential for your safe pregnancy and health of your baby.

- **Smoker? Try to quit:**

Smoking raises the chances of preterm birth, miscarriages, and many serious placental problems. If you continue smoking through your pregnancy, apart from affecting your health, it can cause defects in the development of you baby or still birth (infant birth). Help yourself to stop this smoke entering your baby's lungs.

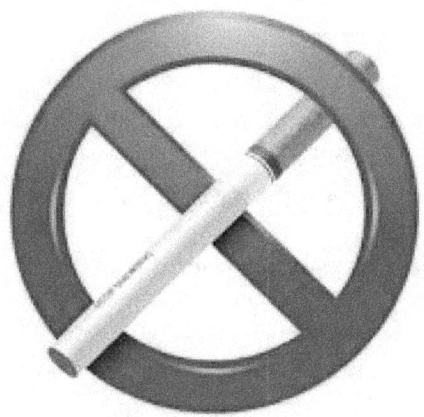

- **Trim back your alcohol:**

Drinking alcohol can cause low birth weight in addition to the defects of speech, language, hearing and thinking of your child. In short, it affects your little one's brain. Alcohol can cross placental barrier, which is there to check the entry of ingredients. Crossing the barrier, it enters the baby's brain and can cause retardation known as fetal alcohol syndrome.

- **Trim back your caffeine:**

Caffeine interferes with the absorption of iron and iron is vital for your pregnancy. So it is recommended to limit your caffeine use. But you can still enjoy your one cup of coffee a day. Limit your use to 200mg of coffee, which is 2 cups of instant coffee a day.

- **Check your medicines:**

Certain medicines can cross placental barrier and can cause harm to the baby. Therefore stop taking unnecessary medications. If there is a certain need then do it with the consultation of your midwife or doctor.

- **Say no to raw foods:**

Raw food is a source of bacteria and parasites which can be harmful for your pregnancy. So keep your hands away from raw meat, raw eggs and uncooked fish.

- **Don't go on diet:**

If you are planning to get smart or remain slim throughout your pregnancy then skip this idea and get back to your normal routine. Dieting can lead to iron, folic acid, other vitamins and minerals deficiency in your body. These deficiencies can be potentially harmful for your baby.

- **Cross your legs for high-impact aerobics:**

High-impact activities are like basketball and gymnastics, which should be avoided during pregnancy. Jumping and hopping can also lead to miscarriages. Sports like football should also be stopped for pregnancy as these can cause trauma to the abdomen (belly). If you are a horseback rider or a lover of scuba diving then skip these by-line activities until and unless you have your healthier baby in your hand.

- **Clean your surroundings:**

If you are routinely exposed to an environment that is contaminated with heavy metals or industrial waste then it can be dangerous. Polluted environments increase the chances of miscarriages and other complications. Make changes for it as soon as possible.

Section 3: Get Over Second Trimester

Feeling recovered from the worst ever nausea? If yes, then welcome to the second trimester of pregnancy, the best and the most enjoyable period of pregnancy. It brings a sense of well-being from its start. The time span of the second trimester is from week 13 to week 27. For this trimester, start shopping for your maternity wardrobe, as your baby is very busy in developing his hair, focusing his lenses and ears, and in learning how to kick your belly.

Chapter 1: Feel the Change

For moms to be, the start of the second trimester means more energy and less discomfort and nausea. You will feel free from the nauseated feeling and will enjoy healthy eating. But, still certain symptoms may persist leaving behind the others. You may feel the following changes.

- **Losing waistline:**

You must expect to gain 2 to 4 pounds every month from the start of the second trimester. Forget your slim smart figure and start looking pregnant. The growing belly is due to your expanding uterus that is increasing in size to make room for your baby.

- **Enlarged breasts:**

Give thanks to additional fat accumulating around your breasts in preparation to produce milk. With this increase in size, much of the tenderness, you experienced in last three months, should be wiped out.

- **Bleeding gums:**

As pregnancy hormones increase circulation, more blood runs through your body. In about half of the pregnant ladies, this more blood makes gums tender, swollen and more sensitive causing them to bleed easily. But this is only temporary; your bleeding gums will get back to their normal state after your delivery.

- **Bleeding nose:**

As with the gums, more blood to nasal mucosa thickens the nasal lining. This leads to swelling and congestion.

- **Aching back:**

The extra weight you gained during this time may exert extra pressure on your back causing back pain. It may cause discomfort in certain postures.

- **Leg cramps:**

Leg cramps may panic you at times. Your growing belly is enough to put pressure on your legs. These kinks may strike you at night.

- **Warm-ups:**

Your uterus is building up for the big task ahead. The contractions in your preparing uterus can be teasing for you. These are called 'Braxton Hicks Contractions'. Some call them false contractions before labor.

- **Darkening skin:**

Estrogen and progesterone of pregnancy give a kicking drive to pigment producing cells of skin (melanin). As a result, dark patches may appear on your skin. A dark line may also appear on your belly button. All these changes will fade away by the time your baby is born.

- **Stretch marks:**

Pink or red streaks may appear on your abdomen and thighs during the second trimester of pregnancy. These stretching marks can be itchy sometimes.

- **Vaginal discharge:**

You will notice thin, white acidic discharge on your under garments. This discharge helps to suppress the growth of harmful bacteria in the uterus and vagina.

- **Life inside you:**

In your first trimester, your baby grows silently inside you. Now be ready to feel the fluttering movements of your baby in your belly. It will move around inside you. This is called 'quickening'. If you don't feel these movements, then don't worry some women don't feel these until the third trimester.

- **Hair growth:**

Pregnancy hormones may boost hair growth along your hairline. Your hair will start shining and flowing.

- **Changes in emotions:**

Increase in weight, cramping legs and aching back all make you feel down and worried all the time. You may feel like crying and have headaches, as well.

Chapter 2: Vitals of the Second Trimester

While enjoying this trimester, set your to-do list for these three months. In the following lines, we give you some tasks for your fitness.

- **Set your appointment with your midwife:**

During the second trimester, arrange your sitting with your caregiver once every four weeks. Your doctor will ask you for an anomaly scan and check your blood pressure.

- **Choose your exercise plan:**

You need to make the most of this energizing period of pregnancy. You can opt for the following exercises in your spare time.

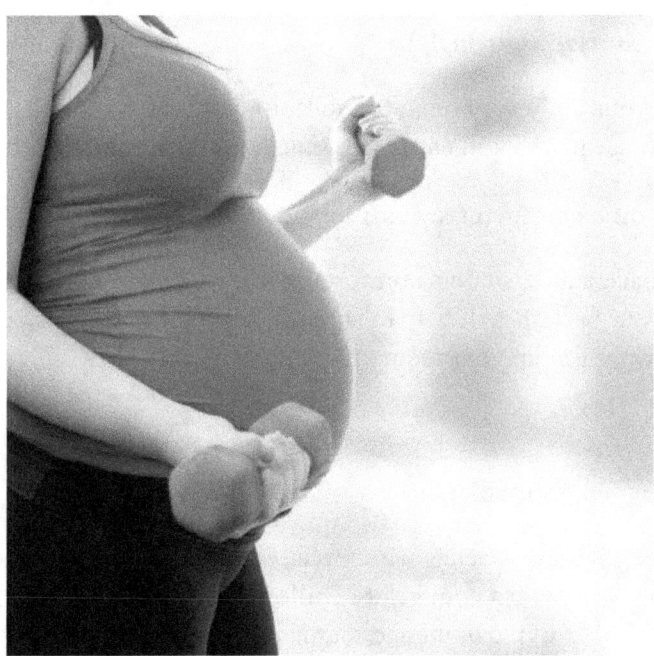

- **Lifting light:**

Light weight for contracting your triceps and biceps will also be interesting for you.

- **Walking track:**

You can walk for 15 to 20 minutes a day to keep yourself fit and healthy.

- **Chair cycle:**

Sitting lazily on the chair? Then play cycling in air with your legs.

- **Kegel exercise:**

Sit comfortably on a chair. Contract your pelvic floor muscle tightly and hold for 10 seconds. It is helpful for contracting the uterus.

- **Take plenty of water:**

Increase your fluid intake to stay hydrated. Take 8 to 10 glasses of water every day. Try carrying a water bottle with you all the time. This water helps to carry essential nutrients through your blood to your baby.

- **Moisturize your belly:**

Moisturize your belly very often to prevent itching of scar marks, as scratching these marks will cause permanent scars on the skin.

- **Sit on a comfortable chair:**

To reduce back aches, sit on a comfortable chair. You can put a comfy pillow on your back. It will help to support your curve. Don't sit on the ground. Always put up your feet to prevent swelling.

- **Sleep on your side:**

Growing belly and back aches will not let you sleep straight. Make sure to sleep on your side with a comfortable pillow behind you. You will remain turning your sides all the night and that is just normal.

Chapter 3: Diet to Take

As nausea and vomiting of the first trimester has faded away, here we have planned another interesting and healthy meal for you. Our plan for you is to give a diet rich in calcium and vitamin D which are essential for the growth of bones and teeth of your baby. These dishes are also rich in vitamin A and omega 3 fatty acids. Let's set a platter for you.

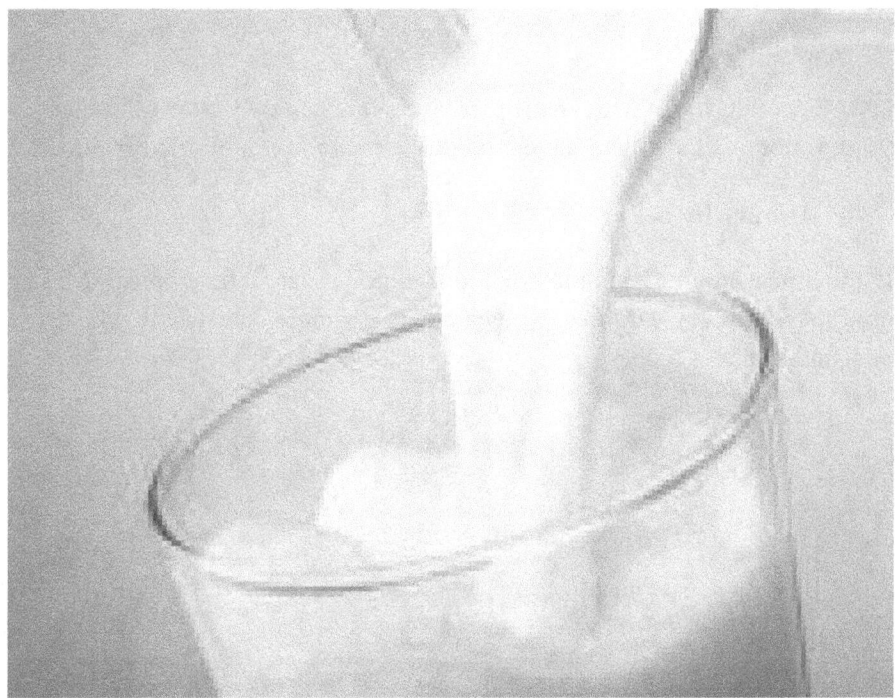

- **Breakfast break:**

As you have survived that bad morning sickness of first trimester, now you can spend a little more time in the kitchen. Try your culinary talent and make something interesting for yourself. For breakfast, you might toast a whole-wheat piece of bread. You can also have eggs, and fruit salad with a glass of milk. For variety, you can mix chopped veggies with an omelet and add some low-fat cheese. A satisfying potato scramble with cheddar cheese can also give you 500 calories.

- **It's snack time:**

In the meanwhile, you can have 1 cup of calcium-fortified skimmed milk full of 90 calories. You can also have kiwi fruit with yogurt

- **Lunch on time:**

Roll Mediterranean salmon salad into a sandwich to get 405 calories. You can also roast chicken with potatoes. If you are still feeling hungry, then don't forget yogurt with a slice of fruit.

- **Again for snack:**

Have vegetable sticks with any dip. You can also enjoy a slice of ginger bread. If not available then have 2 handfuls of walnuts and dried fruits.

- **Dinner by bed:**

By the time of dinner, you may be too tired to prepare a fancy meal. Make some spaghetti with sardines. You can keep it simple with whole wheat pasta and sauce.

Chapter # 4: Don'ts of the Mid Era

You may find yourself battling with a few worries during this trimester. Here is a "don't" list to make you free from those worries.

- **Don't sleep on your back:**

If you are fond of sleeping on your back then it can press your uterus to your spine. This can lead to pain in the lower back and blockage of the blood flow to your baby. It can also cause shortness of breath. Hence it is recommended to sleep on your side. You can even use a pillow below your stomach for some support to your belly.

- **Don't put on high heels:**

You must love to wear a pair of stilettos. As you advance in your pregnancy avoid high heels. Your weight gain and change in body shape changes your balance. This can make it difficult for you to keep your gait steady and you may fall. It is advisable to wear comfy pumps or shoes.

- **Avoid unsafe sports:**

High-impact sports like football, basketball, and horse-riding can throw you in a shell of risk of blow to your belly. Hence it makes sense to avoid such sports.

Section # 4: Count Down To Birth

Third trimester i.e. 28 to 40 weeks must be an exciting yet challenging time for you. You have got only a few weeks to go. We know you are desperately waiting to see the little one in your hands. But, there is a little more to do. In this section, you can find ways to engage yourself for a healthy ride of the third trimester.

Chapter 1: Look Pregnant

Now when you have entered third trimester of pregnancy, you have covered two thirds of your journey. During these days you might desire to hurry things along with your pregnant looking tummy. All the symptoms of pregnancy of the second trimester will follow you here too except, thankfully, nausea.

- **Pregnant belly:**

Your real weight gain starts in these ending weeks. You must have attained 2 to 3 kg by the end of the third trimester. You may be out growing your old wardrobe now. This increase in tummy bulge is your growing uterus because of your busy baby coming to his length.

- **Feeding breast growth:**

With increase in belly, your breasts stay busy in preparing for feeding the new comer. Nipples grow in size and the skin around them becomes darker.

- **Swelling:**

Growing uterus and bulging tummy may exert pressure on the veins returning blood from your feet back to your heart. This causes the swelled feet.

- **Baby you can't sleep:**

Your kicking naughty baby will not let you sleep the whole night. It will feel like floating in your belly full inside of the amniotic fluid. If you can stay asleep the whole night, then relax, you only have a few days to go now.

- **Back with more ache:**

All the increase in your size and shape keeps you're back aching all the time. Your hand will always be there on your back towards the end.

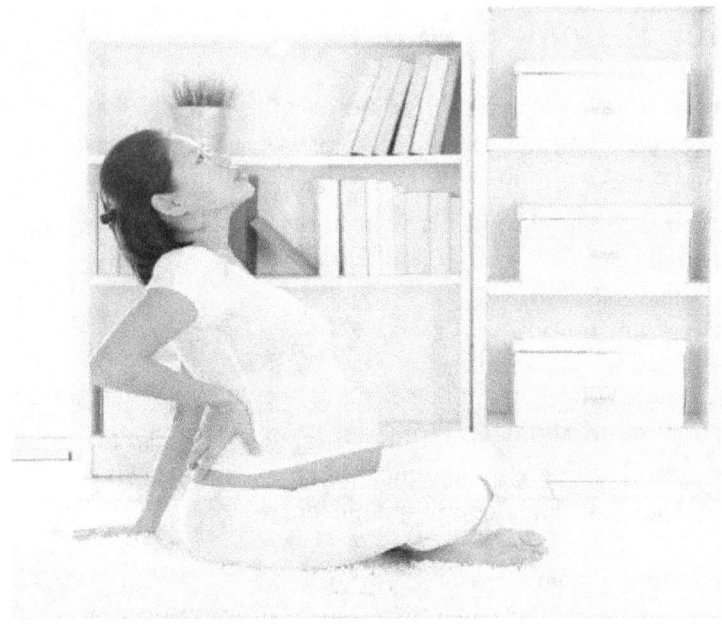

- **Preparing for contractions:**

Braxton hick's contractions that you have felt during the second trimester will get high in intensity. These are false pains preparing you for the final labor for delivery.

Chapter 2: Points to Follow

You already have started counting the days, but besides waiting, do some engaging activities to keep yourself distracted from the end day efforts. Don't think of leaving all the healthy activities of the first and second trimesters during this period. Keep on having fluid intake, relaxing sleep, and a fresh diet. Keep on enjoying your old routine with a little additional to-do list.

- **Massage your bump:**

As your tummy grows in size, you may spend some time thinking on your unborn baby. It's perfectly safe to massage your abdomen for itchy stretch marks. Take out some time for a relaxing massage for your uterus.

- **Do some stretches:**

Third trimester exercises can be very effort putting for you as your body is heavy. Even stretching your shoulders and moving an arm may feel like too much work. But a little exercise is necessary during this period to keep you energetic and fresh.

- **Sleeping stretch pose:**

Lie on your back with the fingers of both hands interlocked. Place these locked hands beneath the head. Bend knees with the soles of your feet on the floor. Move head in either direction.

- **Lying cycling:**

Lie down on the mat. Try air cycling with both legs. Do it slowly. Don't make it a strenuous effort as it will cause shortness of breath.

- **Hunker down:**

Doing squats is the best act you can do for the third trimester. Sit on your heels. Bend your knees and support your hands on a wall or a chair. This will help to broaden the pelvis and ease the delivery of your new comer. Don't squat for more than 10 minutes at a time; it will cause swelling of your feet. Practice 3 times a day.

Chapter 3: Diet to Take

Eating well is always difficult when you are not in a good mood. Your increasing weight may make you somewhat touchy or irritated. But, to have complete healthy food, is essential for the growth of your baby. Therefore, you should choose a nutrient rich food that he or she needs to grow. In our meal plan, we have selected protein rich food for you.

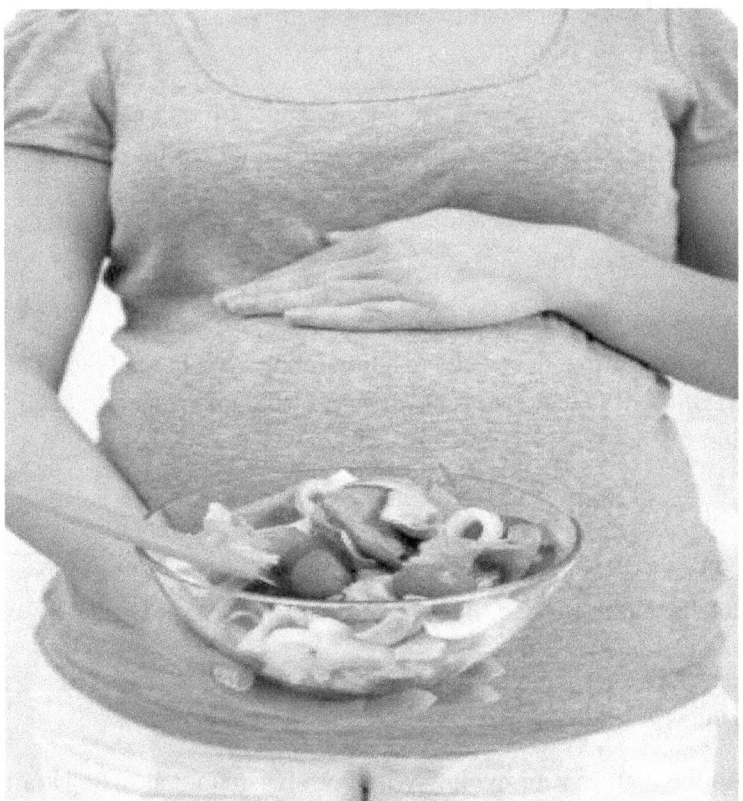

- **Start your morning:**

In the third trimester, you may find yourself exhausted and unable to stay standing for a long time. So give ease to your body and make an easy cheese omelet for your morning. Also have a glass of apple or pineapple juice with it.

- **Snack it:**

Feeling hungry before lunch? Have some melon slices with blueberries and yogurt.

- **Lunch after brunch:**

For lunch, you can roast beef or lamb with roasted potatoes and green beans. If craving a dessert then have some chopped mango.

- **Snack it again:**

Have ½ cup of dried apricot and crunchy walnuts. If you need more of a snack then yogurt will suffice.

- **Dine-in dinner:**

Try creamy chickpea curry for dinner. If you are a rice lover then make egg fried rice too. Don't forget to have calcium-rich milk before going to bed.

Chapter 4: Don'ts Towards the End

By this time you must be busy in narrowing down the baby name's lists and jotting down your pregnancy dreams. But make your mind conscious too of the precautions that you are practicing since the first day of pregnancy.

- **Stay away from teasers:**

Keep stress away from you. Don't panic on old wives' tales of their pregnancy experience. Don't be afraid of labor and the efforts of delivery. Just give peace to your mind and enjoy each and every moment of this blessed journey.

- **Don'ts since the first trimester:**

If you have stopped your bad habits of smoking and alcohol since the first trimester, then it is good for you. If not, then definitely start now. Also stay away from strenuous sports and activities.

- **Stop uplifting:**

Don't try to lift heavy objects, as it can result into miscarriages. Lifting heavy objects can cause imbalance of your posture and lethal results will follow.

Conclusion

If you follow these tips, you can hopefully have an easier pregnancy. We have included several recipes and exercises to make the next nine months as easy as possible. So kick back and relax, and wait for your little bundle of joy.

Author Bio

Muhammad Usman is a distinguished medical graduate of Allama Iqbal medical college (AIMC). He is a professional writer who has been in the field for more than 4 years. During this time he has produced 10,000+ articles, blogs and eBooks on various niches related to diseases, health, fitness, nutrition and well-being. He is a regular contributor to several journals related to medicine and surgery. He is the editor of several journals and newspapers.

Check out some of the other JD-Biz Publishing books
Gardening Series on Amazon

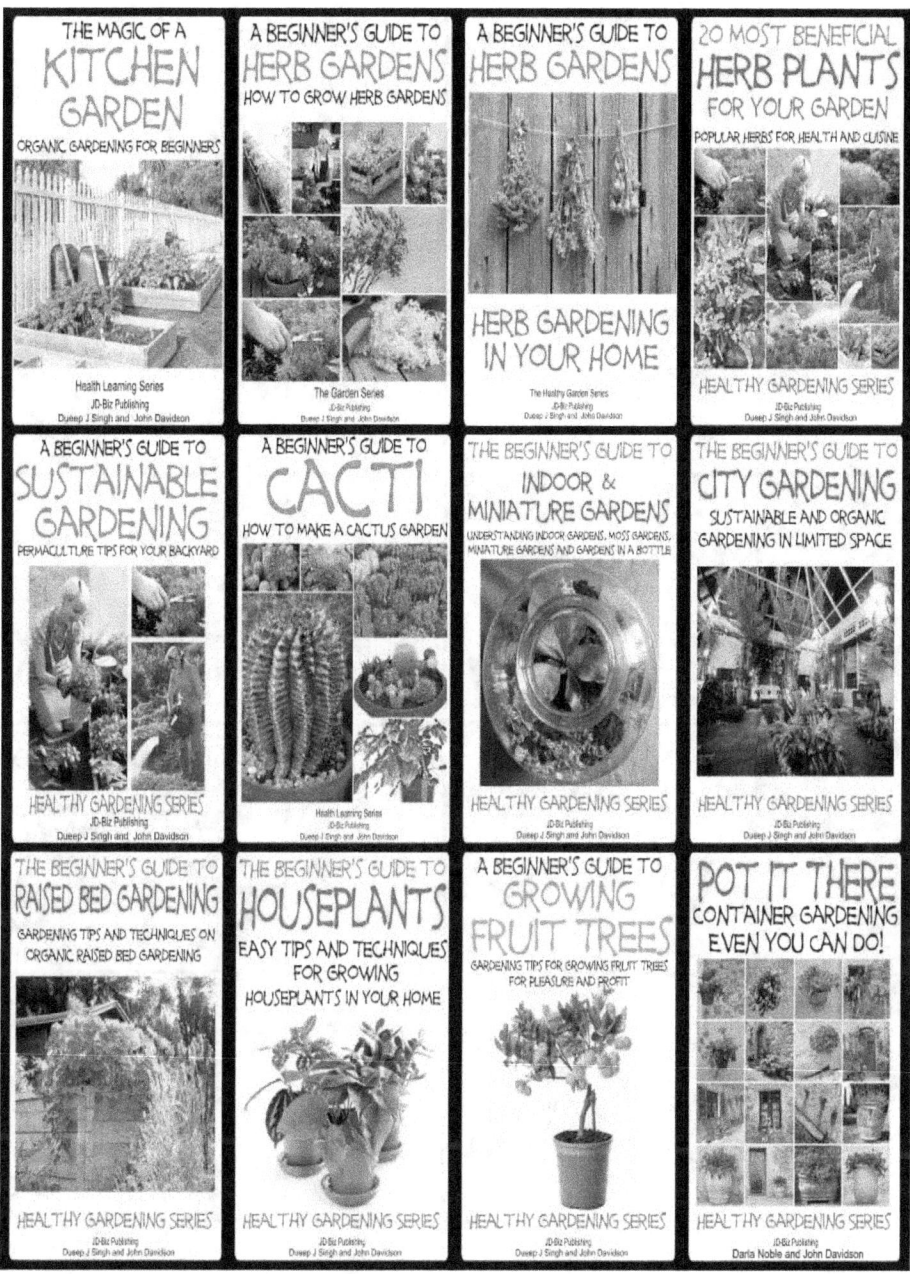

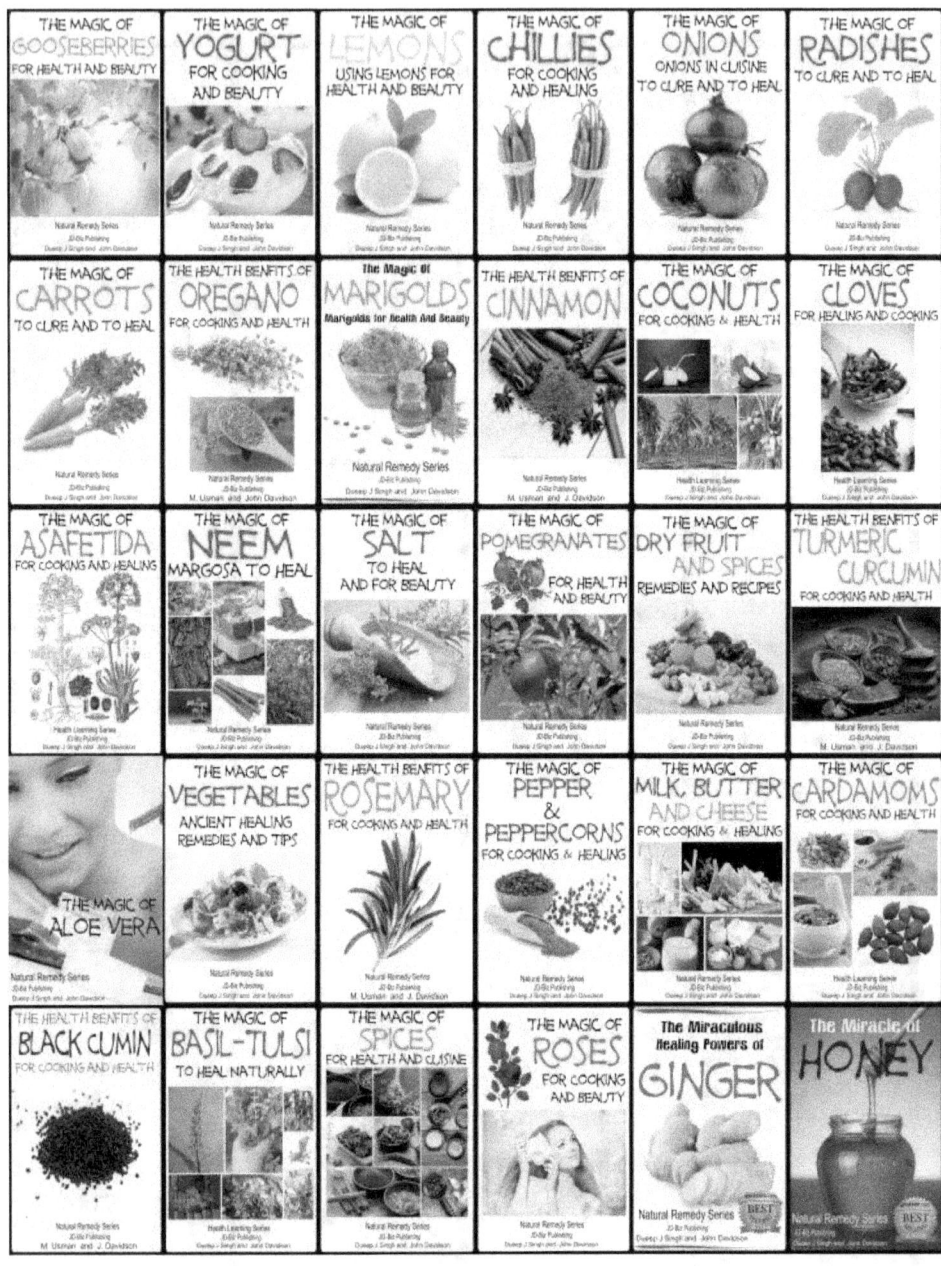

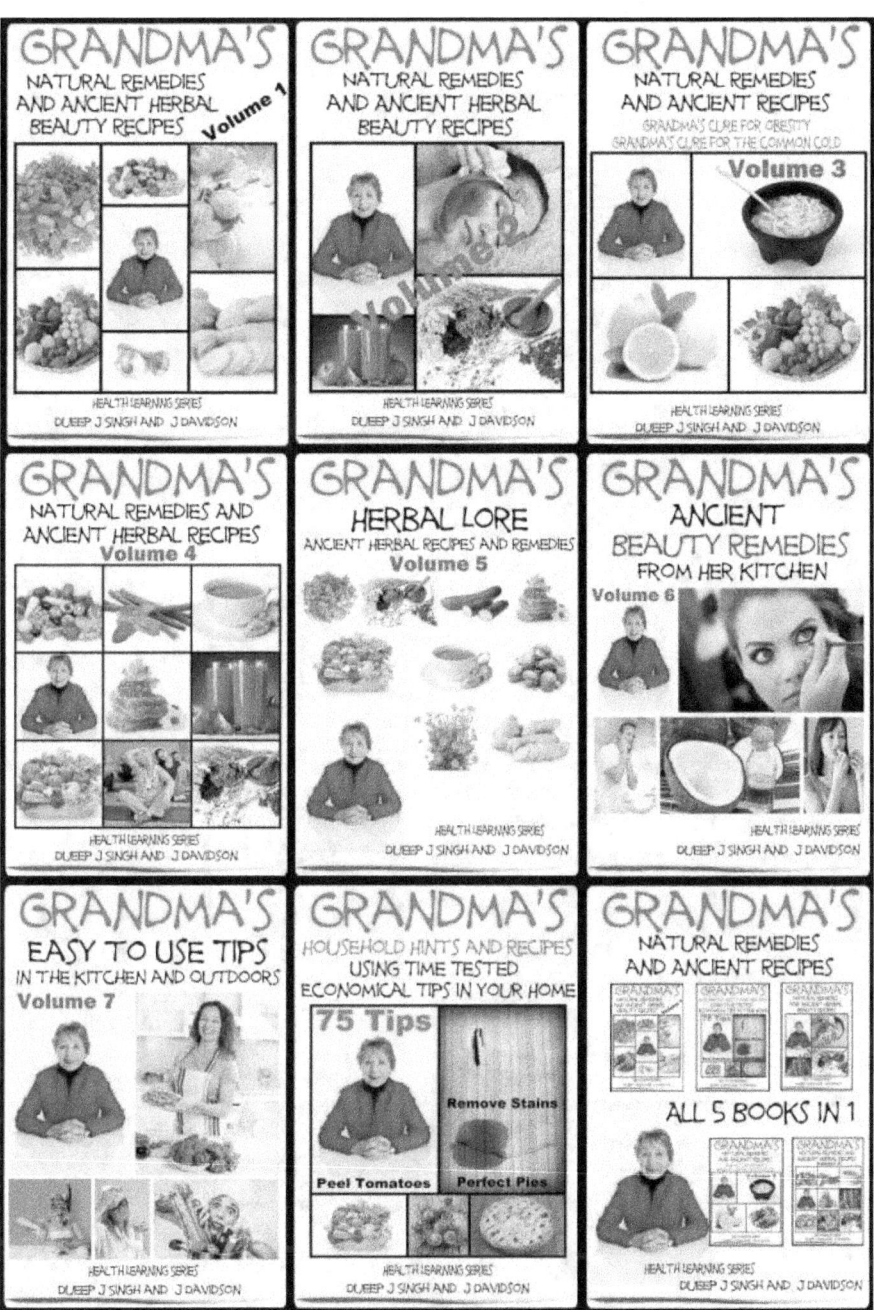

Country Life Books

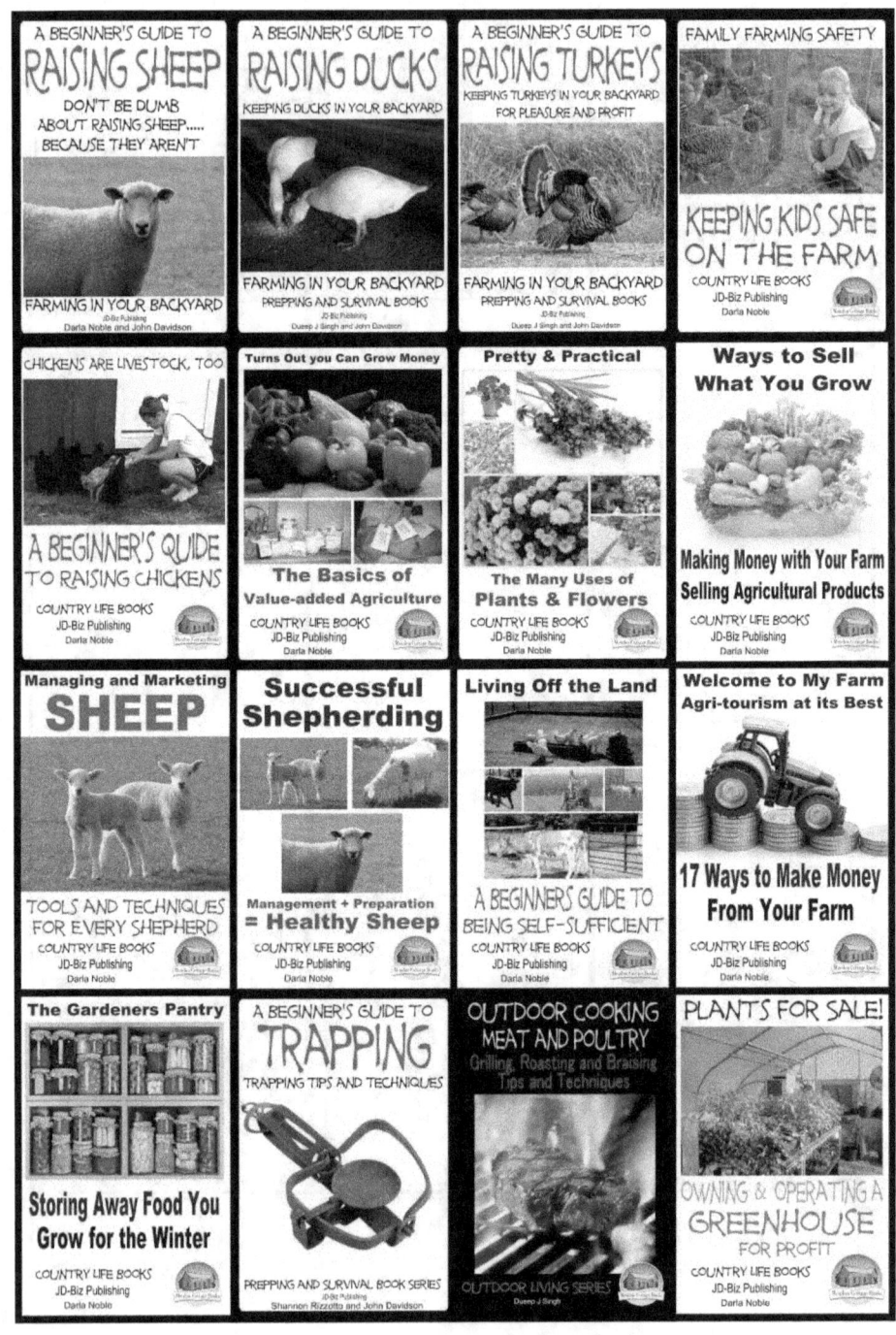

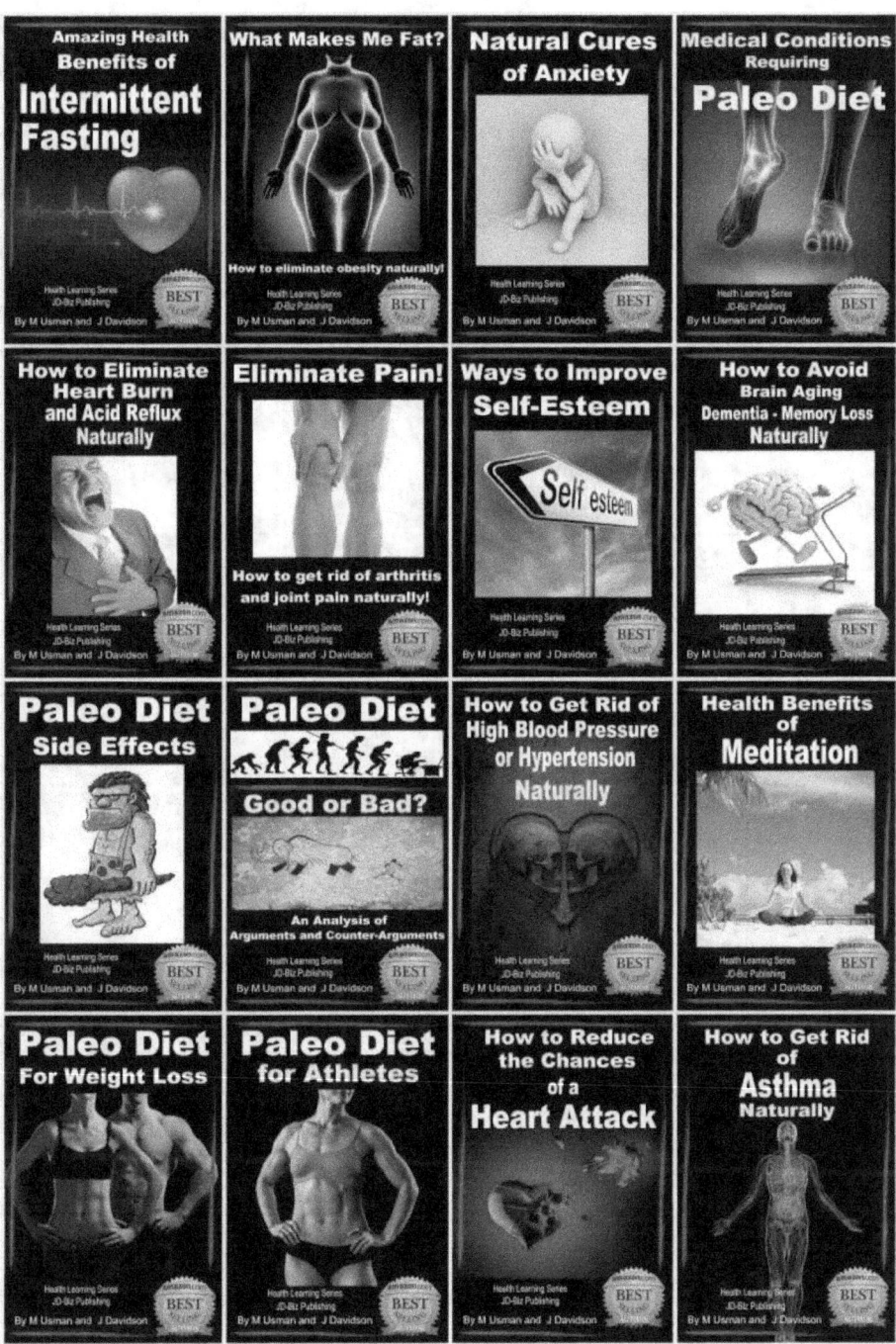

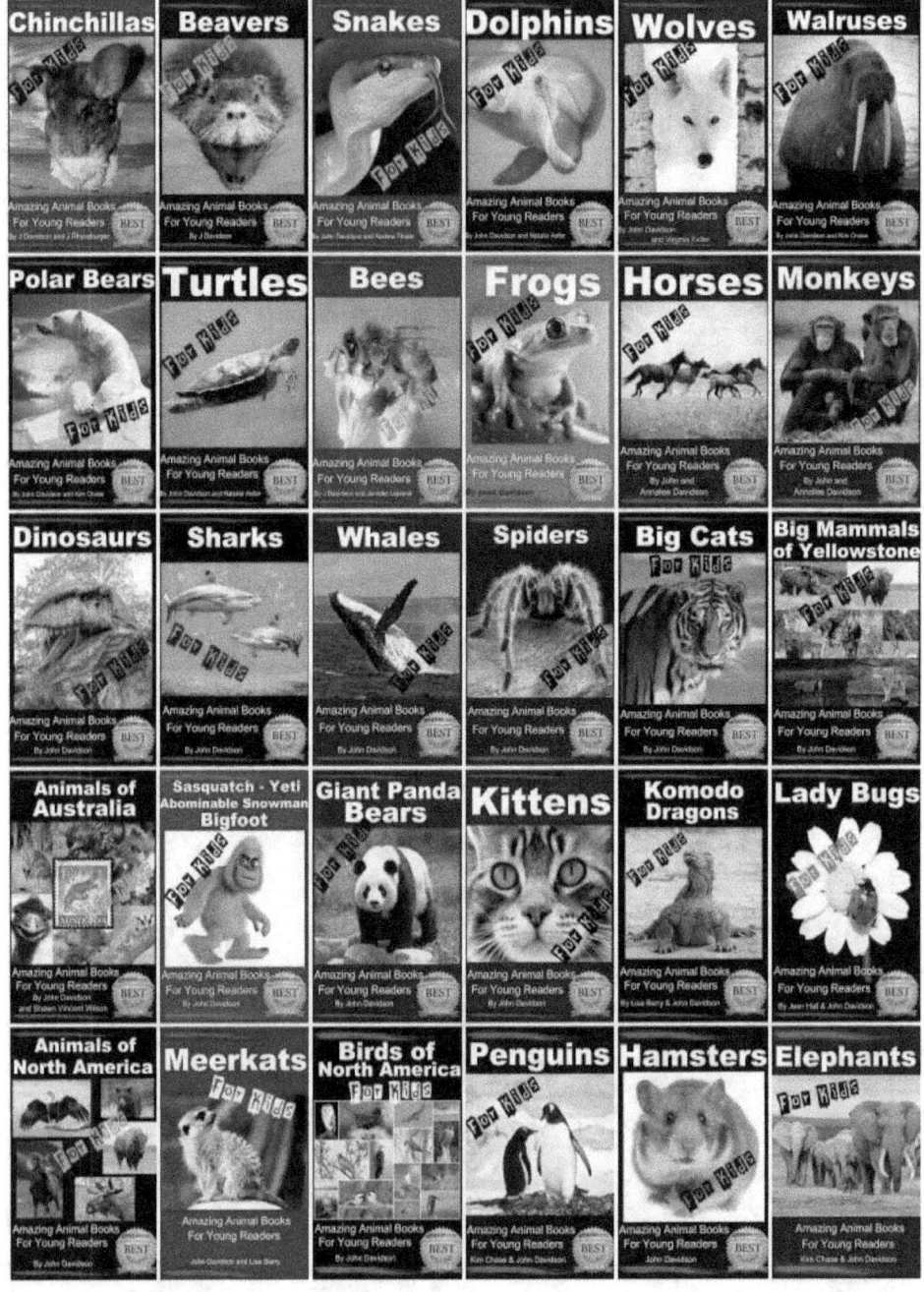

Learn To Draw Series

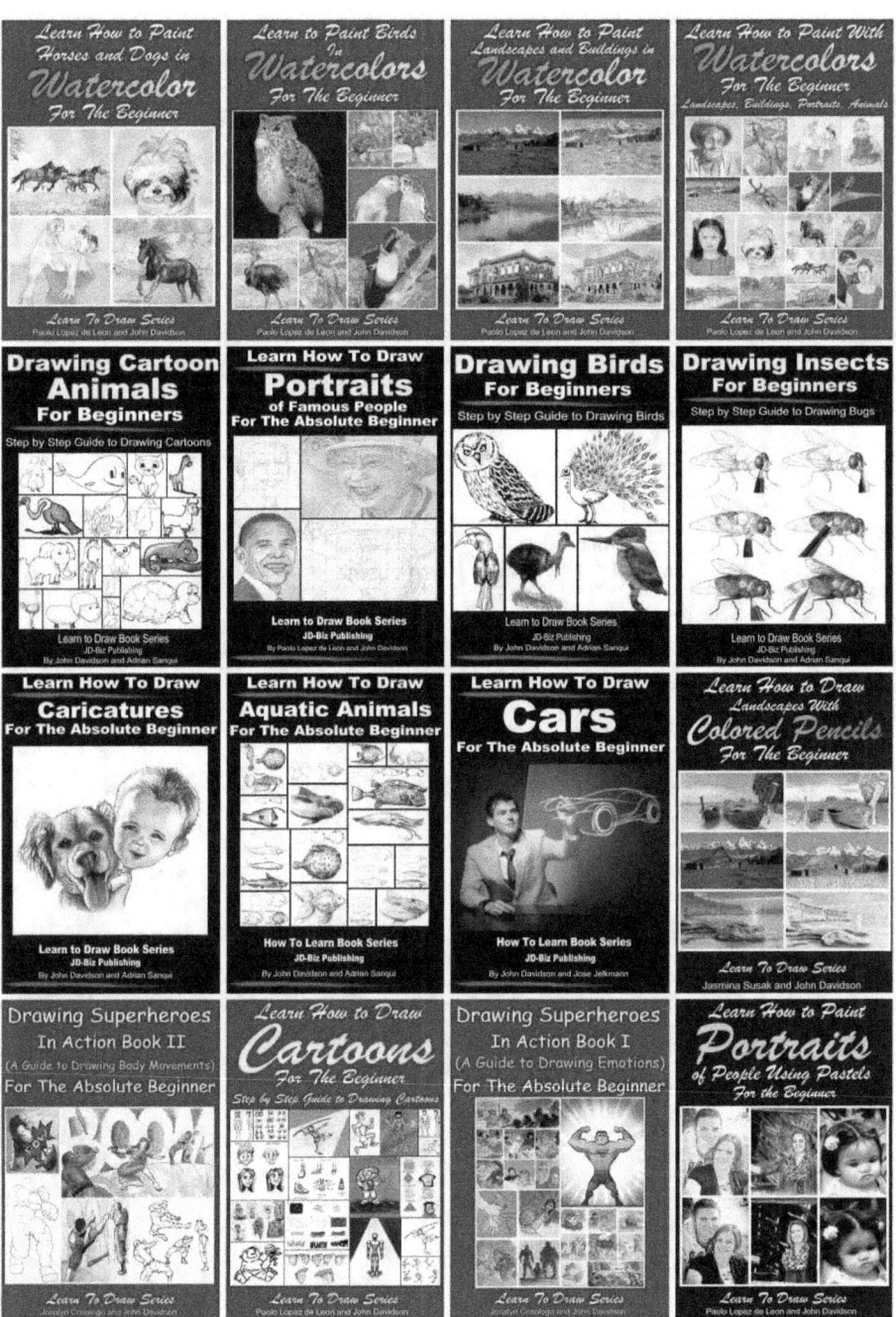

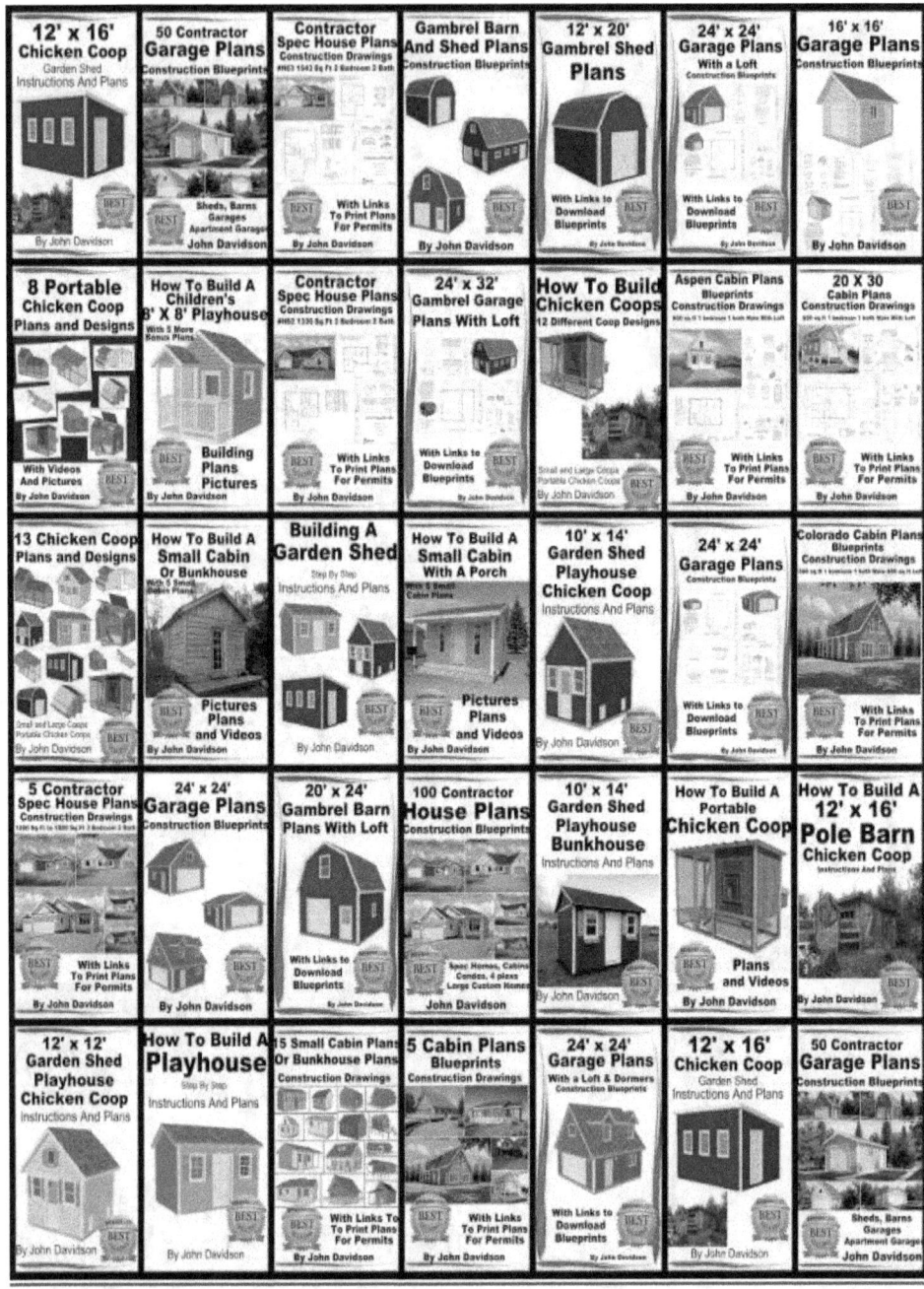

Entrepreneur Book Series

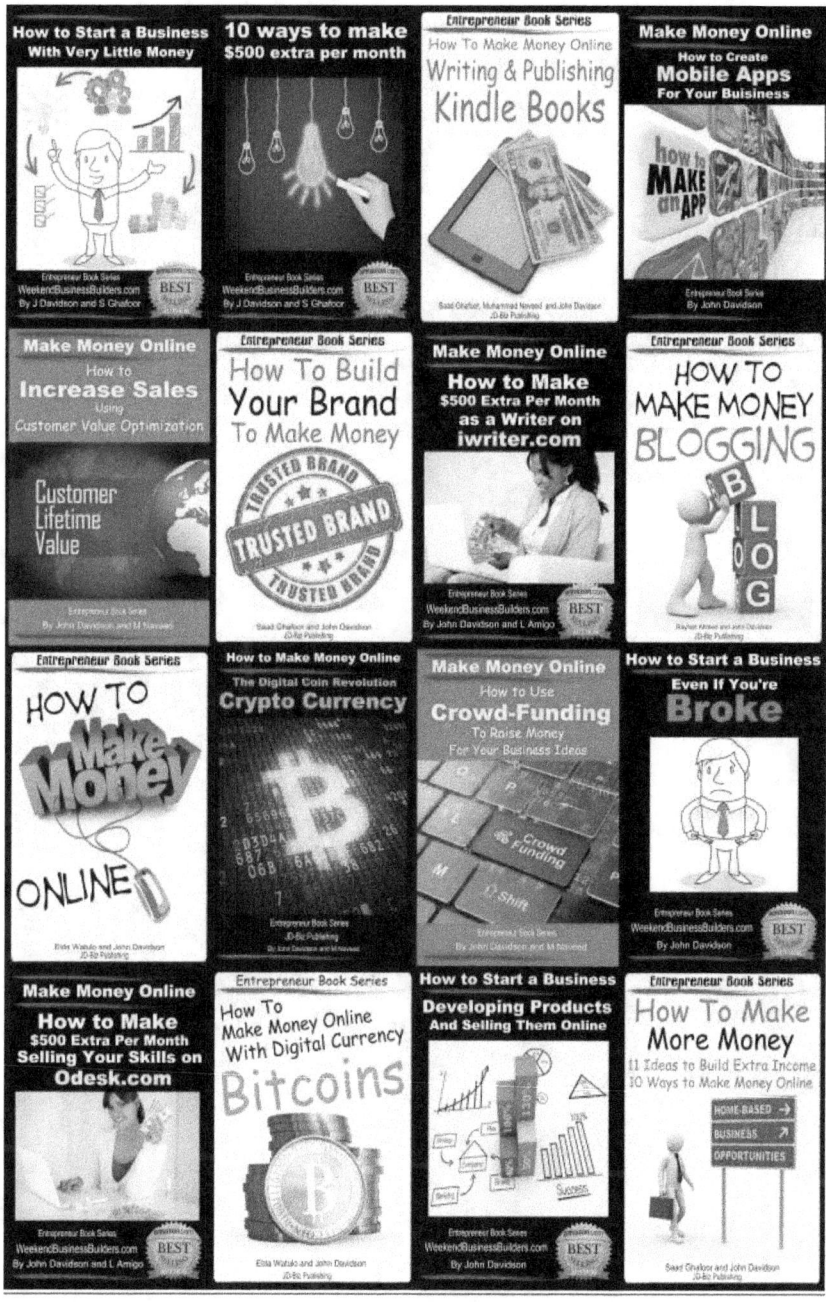

Our books are available at

1. Amazon.com

2. Barnes and Noble

3. Itunes

4. Kobo

5. Smashwords

6. Google Play Books

Publisher

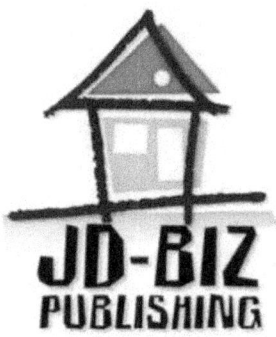

JD-Biz Corp

P O Box 374

Mendon, Utah 84325

http://www.jd-biz.com/

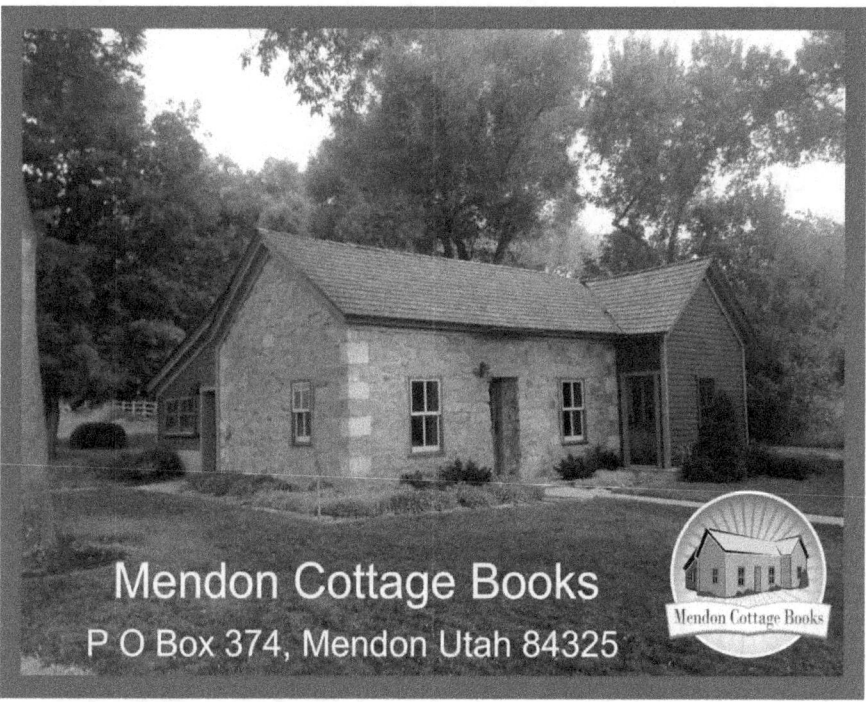

Mendon Cottage Books
P O Box 374, Mendon Utah 84325